LOW SODIUM COOKBOOK

MAIN COURSE - 60+ Breakfast, Lunch, Dinner and Dessert Recipes for Low Sodium Diet

TABLE OF CONTENTS

Introduction

Low Sodium recipes for personal enjoyment but also for family enjoyment. You will love them for sure for how easy it is to prepare them.

BREAKFAST

EGGS AND SPINACH

Serves: *4*

Prep Time: *5*   Minutes

Cook Time: *10*   Minutes

Total Time: *15*   Minutes

INGREDIENTS

- 1 ½ tsp chilli flakes
- 4 eggs
- 3 ½ oz spinach
- 1 lb tomatoes

DIRECTIONS

1. Wilt the spinach
2. Squeeze the excess water out
3. Divide among 4 bowls
4. Mix the tomatoes with the seasoning and chilli flakes
5. Add to the spinach bowls
6. Crack an egg into each bowl and bake for about 15 minutes in the preheated oven at 365F

MORNING SAUSAGE

Serves: **4**

Prep Time: **15**   Minutes

Cook Time: **35**   Minutes

Total Time: **50**   Minutes

INGREDIENTS

- 1 lb ground chicken
- 1 ½ tsp smoked paprika
- ½ tsp salt
- 1 ½ tsp rubbed sage
- 1/3 tsp white pepper
- 1/3 tsp thyme
- 1/5 tsp nutmeg
- 1 ½ tbs olive oil

DIRECTIONS

1. Mix the sage, ground meet, paprika, white pepper, nutmeg, thyme and salt
2. Form patties and place them on a baking sheet
3. Fry the patties in hot oil until brown on both sides
4. Serve immediately

BREAKFAST TACO

Serves: **2**

Prep Time: **10**   Minutes

Cook Time: **20**   Minutes

Total Time: **30**   Minutes

INGREDIENTS

- ¼ cup onion
- 1/3 cup green pepper
- 2 tsp sage
- Corn tortillas
- 1 lb turkey
- 1 tsp thyme
- 4 cups eggs
- 2 lb hash browns

DIRECTIONS

1. Mix hash browns and oil, then spread on a baking pan
2. Bake for about 20 minutes until browned
3. Scramble the eggs with onions and peppers
4. Combine the sage and thyme together

5. Fill a tortilla with ½ cup mixture, then microwave for about 15 seconds

6. Serve immediately

STUFFED POTATOES

Serves: **6**

Prep Time: **10**   Minutes

Cook Time: **20**   Minutes

Total Time: **30**   Minutes

INGREDIENTS

- 3 potatoes
- 1/3 cup scallions
- 3 eggs
- 1/3 tsp salt
- 3 tbs butter
- 1/3 tsp pepper
- ½ cup cheese
- ½ cup red pepper

DIRECTIONS

1. Prick potatoes with a fork and microwave for a few minutes until tender
2. Cut the potatoes lengthwise and scoop out the flesh
3. Cook the bell pepper, scallions and chopped potato flesh in melted butter for about 3 minutes

4. Add eggs, salt and pepper and cook 2 more minutes
5. Remove from heat and fold in the cheese
6. Stuff each potato half with the mixture, allow to cool and wrap with foil
7. Refrigerate overnight
8. Cook for about 10 minutes turning once
9. Serve immediately

AVOCADO TOAST

Serves:	*2*	
Prep Time:	*5*	Minutes
Cook Time:	*5*	Minutes
Total Time:	*10*	Minutes

INGREDIENTS
Pesto:
- 1 ½ tbs olive oil
- 1 tbs hot water
- 1/8 tsp black pepper
- ¼ tsp garlic powder
- 1/3 cup basil leaves
- ¼ cup walnuts
- 1 lemon

Toast:
- 1/3 tsp black pepper
- 2 tsp olive oil
- 4 slices bread
- 1 avocado

DIRECTIONS

1. Place the pesto ingredients into a food processor and pulse until smooth
2. Toast the bread
3. Divide the avocado slices
4. Spread pesto over avocado, then drizzle with lemon juice and olive oil
5. Serve immediately

Serves: **12**
Prep Time: **10**   Minutes

Cook Time: **30**   Minutes

Total Time: **40**   Minutes

INGREDIENTS

- 4 eggs
- 3 cups hash brown
- 12 oz turkey sausage
- 1 bell pepper
- 1 cup cheese
- 2 cups milk
- 1 onion
- ½ tsp salt
- ¼ tsp black pepper

DIRECTIONS

1. Cook the onion, pepper and sausage until done
2. Stir together with frozen potatoes and ½ cup cheese, then place into a baking dish

3. Mix together milk, pepper, salt and eggs and pour over

4. Bake uncovered for about 30 minutes

5. Sprinkle with cheese and bake 2 more minutes

6. Allow to cool, then serve

HAM OMELETTE

Serves: **2**
Prep Time: **10**   Minutes

Cook Time: **20**   Minutes

Total Time: **30**   Minutes

INGREDIENTS

- 4 eggs
- 1 tbs paprika
- 2 tbs olive oil
- ½ tbs onion powder
- ½ cup onion
- 1/3 cup ham
- ½ cup red pepper
- ½ tbs garlic powder

DIRECTIONS

1. Sauté the onion in hot oil
2. Add in the red pepper and sauté until roasted on edges
3. Add ham and paprika and cook 2 more minutes
4. Whisk together the eggs in a bowl

5. Scramble the eggs in hot oil in another skillet

6. Sprinkle with onion and garlic powder

7. Place the ham mixture on one half of the omelette and fold it

8. Serve immediately

QUICHE CUPS

Serves: *8*
Prep Time: *10*   Minutes

Cook Time: *30*   Minutes

Total Time: *40*   Minutes

INGREDIENTS

- 10 oz broccoli
- 2 drops hot sauce
- 1/3 tsp black pepper
- 4 eggs
- 1 cup cheese
- ½ cup bell peppers
- 1 green onion

DIRECTIONS

1. Squeeze the vegetables dry
2. Blend the ingredients together using a food processor
3. Divide among a lined muffin pan
4. Bake for about 30 minutes
5. Allow to cool, then serve

CHICKEN SAUSAGE

Serves: **4**

Prep Time: **5**   Minutes

Cook Time: **10**   Minutes

Total Time: **15**   Minutes

INGREDIENTS

- ½ tsp red pepper flakes
- 1 ½ tsp maple syrup
- 3 tsp olive oil
- 1 ½ tsp sage
- 1 ½ tsp garlic powder
- 1 ½ tsp black pepper
- 1 lb. ground chicken

DIRECTIONS

1. Mix everything together except for the oil
2. Form patties from the mixture
3. Cook the patties in hot oil until cooked through
4. Serve immediately

BURRITO BOWL

Serves: **4**

Prep Time: **10**   Minutes

Cook Time: **15**   Minutes

Total Time: **25**   Minutes

INGREDIENTS

- 2 tbs olive oil
- ½ cup almond milk
- 2 tbs shallot
- 1 cup red pepper
- 1/3 cup salsa
- 2 eggs
- 2 egg whites
- ½ cup onion
- 2 avocados
- 15 oz pinto beans
- 2 tsp cumin
- 1 cup cherry tomatoes

DIRECTIONS

1. Sauté the onion until soft
2. Add the red peppers and cook until they are also soft
3. Add chili powder, pinto beans and cumin, cook a little more, then cover and turn the heat off
4. Chop the tomatoes and avocados
5. Combine ½ chopped avocado, shallot, salsa and almond milk in a food processor
6. Pulse until combined
7. Scramble the eggs and egg whites
8. Divide the bean mixture into bowls, top with avocado, tomatoes, eggs and drizzle with avocado sauce
9. Serve immediately

LUNCH MEATLOAF

Serves: *8*

Prep Time: *10*   Minutes

Cook Time: *60*   Minutes

Total Time: *70*   Minutes

INGREDIENTS

Meatloaf:
- 2 tbs olive oil
- ½ cup carrot
- 2 lbs ground beef
- ½ cup celery
- 1 cup oats
- 2 tbs Worcestershire sauce
- 1/3 cup milk
- 2 tsp seasoning mix
- 1 egg
- 2 tsp garlic
- ½ cup onion
- 1 tsp black pepper

Sauce:

- 8 oz tomato sauce
- 2 tbs mustard
- 2 tbs vinegar
- 1/3 cup brown sugar

DIRECTIONS

1. Sauté the carrot, celery and onion in olive oil
2. Mix the meatloaf ingredients together and place in a baking pan
3. Mix the sauce ingredients together and pour over the meatloaf
4. Bake in the preheated oven for about 1 hour at 350F

TURKEY WRAP

Serves: *1*
Prep Time: *5*   Minutes

Cook Time: *10*   Minutes

Total Time: *15*   Minutes

INGREDIENTS

- 2 slices turkey breast
- 2 slices ham
- 1 tsp mustard
- 1 tsp mayonnaise
- 1 tortilla wrap
- 1/3 cup arugula

DIRECTIONS

1. Mix the mayonnaise and mustard together, then spread on the tortilla
2. Place the arugula over, then add the ham and turkey slices
3. Roll up the wrap
4. Serve immediately

LUNCH RAMEN

Serves: *1*

Prep Time: *5*   Minutes

Cook Time: *10*   Minutes

Total Time: *15*   Minutes

INGREDIENTS

- 1 tsp bullion
- 1/3 cup dehydrated vegetables
- 1 cup noodles

DIRECTIONS

1. Place the ingredients in a jar
2. Fill with water and microwave for 3 minutes

LETTUCE WRAPS

Serves: **4**

Prep Time: **5**   Minutes

Cook Time: **10**   Minutes

Total Time: **15**   Minutes

INGREDIENTS
Sauce:
- 2 limes
- 1 ½ tsp cornstarch
- 2 tbs water
- 5 tbs soy sauce
- 2 tbs ginger
- 1 tbs vinegar
- 3 cloves garlic
- 2 tbs honey
- 2 tbc chili paste

Chicken:
- 3 green onions
- 1/3 cup cashews
- 16 lettuce leaves

- 2 tbs olive oil
- 1 lb ground chicken

DIRECTIONS

1. Mix the sauce ingredients together and stir to combine
2. Cook the chicken in hot oil until browned
3. Add the cashews and cook for another 2 minutes
4. Add the sauce and cook 2 more minutes
5. Stir in the green onions and remove from heat
6. Place the mixture onto each lettuce leaf, then roll up
7. Serve immediately

VEGETABLE SOUP

Serves: *10*

Prep Time: *10*   Minutes

Cook Time: *20*   Minutes

Total Time: *30*   Minutes

INGREDIENTS

- 1 onion
- 1 cup carrots
- 5 cups cabbage
- 1 cup green beans
- 3 cloves garlic
- 1 tsp basil
- Black pepper
- 3 tbs tomato paste
- 3 bay leaves
- 1 tsp thyme
- 2 bell peppers
- 1 can tomatoes
- 5 cups beef broth
- 2 cup broccoli
- 2 cups zucchini

DIRECTIONS

1. Cook the garlic and onion until soft
2. Add the cabbage, carrots and green beans and cook 5 more minutes
3. Add the tomatoes, tomato paste, broth, bell peppers, bay leaves, and seasoning
4. Simmer for 5 minutes
5. Add in the zucchini and broccoli and simmer for 5 more minutes
6. Remove bay leaves and serve

CHICKEN AND BROCCOLI

Serves: **4**

Prep Time: **5**   Minutes

Cook Time: **10**   Minutes

Total Time: **15**   Minutes

INGREDIENTS

- 1 lb chicken thighs
- 1 ½ tbs sesame seeds
- 2 tsp garlic
- 1/3 cup oyster sauce
- 2 tbs oil
- 1/3 cup chicken broth
- 2 tsp honey
- 1 tsp sesame oil
- 2 cups broccoli florets
- 1 ½ tsp soy sauce
- 1 tsp cornstarch
- Salt
- Pepper

DIRECTIONS

1. Cook the broccoli in hot oil until tender
2. Add the garlic and cook 30 more seconds
3. Place the seasoned chicken in the pan and cook until browned
4. Mix the oyster sauce, honey, soy sauce, chicken broth and sesame oil together
5. Combine the cornstarch with 1 tbs of cold water
6. Pour the oyster mixture over the chicken and broccoli and cook for 30 seconds
7. Add the cornstarch, bring to a boil and cook for a minute
8. Serve topped with sesame seeds

CHICKEN AND RICE

Serves: **4**

Prep Time: **10** Minutes

Cook Time: **20** Minutes

Total Time: **30** Minutes

INGREDIENTS

- 1 cup rice
- 15 oz salsa
- 3 tsp paprika
- 3 tbs olive oil
- 1 ½ cup chicken broth
- 2 lb chicken thigh

DIRECTIONS

1. Cut the chicken and toss with the paprika
2. Cook in hot oil until browned
3. Add the rice and mix well, cooking 1 more minute to toast the rice
4. Add the broth and salsa and stir
5. Bring to a simmer, then cover and cook for 20 minutes
6. Serve immediately

EASY TACOS

Serves: **8**

Prep Time: **10** Minutes

Cook Time: **20** Minutes

Total Time: **30** Minutes

INGREDIENTS

- Tortilla shells
- 3 bell peppers
- 2 tbs olive oil
- 2 cups green lentils
- 1 onion
- 3 cloves garlic
- 3 cups mushrooms
- 1 package taco seasoning
- 2 tsp paprika
- 1 cup water
- Parsley

DIRECTIONS

1. Sauté the peppers in hot oil until soft

2. Add the onions and garlic and cook until soft
3. Add the mushrooms, lentils, paprika and taco seasoning and stir until the mushrooms release some juice
4. Add the water slowly to create a sauce
5. Reduce the heat and cook for 15 minutes
6. Add the bell peppers and combine
7. Place the mixture onto each taco shell
8. Serve immediately

BBQ CHICKEN

Serves: **4**

Prep Time: **10**   Minutes

Cook Time: **5**   Hours

Total Time: **40**   Minutes

INGREDIENTS

- 1/3 cup chicken broth
- 1 cup BBQ sauce
- 1 ½ lbs chicken breasts

DIRECTIONS

1. Place the ingredients in a crockpot and cook on low for 5 hours
2. Break the meat to shred
3. Serve over a bun

TUNA MELTS

Serves: 2
Prep Time: 5   Minutes
Cook Time: 5   Minutes
Total Time: 10   Minutes

INGREDIENTS

- 6 oz tuna
- 3 tbs onion
- ¼ tsp salt
- ¼ tsp black pepper
- 1 avocado
- 3 tbs Greek yogurt
- 3 oz cheese
- 2 tomatoes

DIRECTIONS

1. Mix together onion, tuna, diced avocado, Greek yogurt, salt, and pepper
2. Place tomato slices on a baking sheet on a wire rack
3. To each slice with tuna mixture, then top with cheese
4. Broil until cheese is melted

SALADS

FRESH SALAD

Serves: **1**

Prep Time: **5** Minutes

Cook Time: **5** Minutes

Total Time: **10** Minutes

INGREDIENTS

- 1 lb beef
- 1 package taco seasoning
- 1 iceberg lettuce
- 3 tomatoes
- 1 cup cheese
- 1/3 cup corn
- 1 bunch scallions

DIRECTIONS

1. Brown the beef, then season
2. In a bowl mix all ingredients and mix well
3. Serve with dressing

Serves: **6**

Prep Time: **5** Minutes

Cook Time: **5** Minutes

Total Time: **10** Minutes

INGREDIENTS

- 3 cups chicken
- 1 cup pecans
- ½ cup Greek yogurt
- 3 celery stalks
- 1/3 cup mayonnaise
- 3 tsp mustard
- 2 tsp vinegar
- 1 tsp salt
- Black pepper
- 1/3 cup red onion
- ¼ cup parsley

DIRECTIONS

1. **Toast the pecans**

2. Cook the chicken
3. Allow the pecans to cool, then chop
4. In a bowl mix all ingredients and mix well
5. Serve with dressing

TUNA SALAD

Serves: *1*
Prep Time: *5*   Minutes

Cook Time: *5*   Minutes

Total Time: *10*   Minutes

INGREDIENTS

- 1 can tuna
- Black pepper
- 3 tbs onion
- 1 pickle
- 2 onions
- ½ rib celery

DIRECTIONS

1. In a bowl mix all ingredients and mix well
2. Serve with romaine lettuce

MEXICAN SALAD

Serves: *1*

Prep Time: **5**   Minutes

Cook Time: **5**   Minutes

Total Time: **10** Minutes

INGREDIENTS
Dressing:
- 5 tbs olive oil
- 1 tsp black pepper
- 2 cloves garlic
- 1 tsp salt
- 1 ½ tsp cumin
- 3 tbs lime juice

Salad:
- 5 tbs salsa
- 5 tbs pumpkin seeds
- 6 cups lettuce
- 1 can corn
- 3 eggs
- 10 oz chicken breast
- 1 can black beans

DIRECTIONS

1. Grill the chicken breast
2. Mix the dressing ingredients together
3. In a separate bowl, mix all the remaining ingredients
4. Serve with dressing

CORN SALAD

Serves: *1*

Prep Time: *5*   Minutes

Cook Time: *5*   Minutes

Total Time: *10*   Minutes

INGREDIENTS

- 5 cups corn
- 3 tomatoes
- 1/3 cup basil
- 1/3 cup olive oil
- 3 tbs vinegar
- Salt
- Pepper
- 1 onion

DIRECTIONS

1. In a bowl mix all ingredients and mix well
2. Serve with dressing

BEAN SALAD

Serves: *1*
Prep Time: *5*   Minutes

Cook Time: *5*   Minutes

Total Time: *10*   Minutes

INGREDIENTS

- 1 cup green beans
- 2 cloves garlic
- 1/3 cup red pepper
- ½ cup red onion
- 15 oz black beans
- 1/3 cup vinegar
- 2 tbs sugar
- 3 tbs oil
- 7 oz red kidney beans
- 1 tsp celery seeds
- 1 tsp dry mustard

DIRECTIONS

1. **Cook the beans**

2. In a bowl mix all ingredients and mix well

3. Serve with dressing made of: sugar, oil, vinegar, dry mustard, celery seeds and garlic

EGG SALAD

Serves: **4**

Prep Time: **5** Minutes

Cook Time: **5** Minutes

Total Time: **10** Minutes

INGREDIENTS

- 2 tbs mustard
- 2 tbs seasoning blend
- 4 eggs
- 3 tbs pickle relish
- 4 tbs mayonnaise
- 1/3 cup celery
- 1/3 cup onion

DIRECTIONS

1. Hard boil the eggs
2. Allow to cool, peel and chop
3. Place everything into a blender and pulse until well mixed
4. Serve cold

APPLE SALAD

Serves: **1**

Prep Time: **5** Minutes

Cook Time: **5** Minutes

Total Time: **10** Minutes

INGREDIENTS

- 1/3 cup apple juice
- 3 tbs lemon juice
- 2 tbs olive oil
- 2 tsp brown sugar
- 1 tsp Dijon mustard
- 1/3 tsp apple pie spice
- 1 apple
- 8 cups salad greens

DIRECTIONS

1. In a bowl mix all ingredients and mix well
2. Serve immediately

AVOCADO SALAD

Serves: **4**

Prep Time: **5**   Minutes

Cook Time: **5**   Minutes

Total Time: **10**   Minutes

INGREDIENTS

- 1/3 cup Greek yogurt
- 2 tbs sour cream
- 1 lime
- 4 eggs
- 1 avocado
- 2 green onions
- 2 tbs dill
- ¼ tsp salt
- ¼ black pepper
- 5 slices bacon

DIRECTIONS

1. Boil the eggs, then peel and dice
2. Mix the dressing ingredients: sour cream, dill, yogurt, lime juice, salt, and pepper

3. In a separate bowl mix all the remaining ingredients
4. Serve with dressing

BLUE CHEESE SALAD

Serves: **12**

Prep Time: **5**   Minutes

Cook Time: **5**   Minutes

Total Time: **10**   Minutes

INGREDIENTS
Salad:
- 2 lb spinach
- 1/3 cup clue cheese
- 1 1/3 cucumbers
- 1 cup tomatoes
- 1/3 cup red onion
- 1/3 cup walnuts

Dressing:
- 5 tbs olive oil
- 1/3 tsp nutmeg
- 3 tbs vinegar
- 1 ½ tbs maple syrup
- 2 tbs yogurt

DIRECTIONS

1. Mix the dressing ingredients together
2. Mix the salad ingredients together
3. Serve with dressing

DINNER

CHICKEN PENNE

Serves: **7**

Prep Time: **10**   Minutes

Cook Time: **60**   Minutes

Total Time: **70**   Minutes

INGREDIENTS
Spices:
- 2 tsp Cumin
- 3 tsp oregano
- 1 tsp onion powder
- 4 tsp chilli powder
- 1 ½ tsp soy flour
- 1 tsp garlic powder
- 1 tsp Cayenne pepper

Chicken:
- 1 ½ lb chicken breast
- 12 oz pasta
- 3 green onions
- 1 cup bell peppers
- 1/3 cup sour cream

- 1 cup cheese
- 3 tomatoes
- 1 1/3 cup milk
- 5 oz cream cheese
- 15 oz black beans

DIRECTIONS

1. Mix the spices together
2. Combine sour cream, milk, cheese, and cream cheese
3. Microwave until soft, then stir in the spices
4. Cook the pasta, then rinse the black beans and pat dry
5. Dice the vegetables and mix with pasta and black beans
6. Add the mixture to a dish and spread out evenly
7. Dice the chicken breast and place on top
8. Pour the cheese sauce over
9. Bake for 30 minutes covered at 360F, then remove cover and bake 30 more minutes at 380
10. Serve immediately

PORK CHOPS

Serves: *3*

Prep Time: *10*   Minutes

Cook Time: *8*   Hours

Total Time: *8*   Hours

INGREDIENTS

- 5 pork loin chops
- 3 cloves garlic
- ½ red onion
- 1 lemon
- 1/8 cup olive oil
- 1/8 cup honey
- 2 tsp oregano
- 2 tsp black pepper

DIRECTIONS

1. Mix lemon zest and lemon juice together along with the remaining ingredients
2. Toss well to coat the pork
3. Refrigerate for about 8 hours

4. Allow the meat to come to room temperature, then grill on a preheated grill pan for about 6 minutes per side

5. Allow to rest, then serve

CHICKEN & MUSHROOM RISOTTO

Serves: *4*

Prep Time: *10*   Minutes

Cook Time: *50*   Minutes

Total Time: *60*   Minutes

INGREDIENTS

- 1 l chicken stock
- 4 tbs P
- armesan
- 2 shallots
- 1 garlic clove
- 2 tbs butter
- 1 can white wine
- ¾ lb mushrooms
- 2 tbs thyme
- 2 tbs olive oil
- 3 chicken breasts
- ½ lb pearl barley

DIRECTIONS

1. Sauté the shallots and garlic with seasoning for 5 minutes in melted butter and oil

2. Stir in the chicken and cook for 3 minutes

3. Add in the barley and cook for another minute

4. Pour in wine and stir until absorbed

5. Add the mushroom and thyme and pour over ¾ of the stock

6. Cook on a low simmer for about 50 minutes

7. Remove from heat and stir in Parmesan

8. Serve immediately

BEEF STROGANOFF

Serves: *6*

Prep Time: *10* Minutes

Cook Time: *30* Minutes

Total Time: *40* Minutes

INGREDIENTS

- 1 lb beef sirloin
- 2 carrots
- 1 ½ tsp black pepper
- 2 tsp mustard
- ¼ cup sour cream
- 1/3 cup red wine
- 1 package noodles
- 6 oz mushrooms
- 3 tbs olive oil
- 2 cup beef stock
- 3 tbs flour
- ½ onion

DIRECTIONS

1. Mix the black pepper and flour together
2. Coat the steak with the mixture
3. Cook the steak in hot oil until browned
4. Cook the mushrooms, carrots and onions for a few minutes until golden brown
5. Turn off the heat and pour in the wine and beef stock
6. Turn up the heat and cook for 3 more minutes
7. Cook the noodles
8. Turn the heat off and mix in the sour cream and mustard
9. Add the beef back and mix to coat
10. Serve the beef mixture over the noodles

JAMAICAN FISH

Serves: **4**

Prep Time: **10** Minutes

Cook Time: **20** Minutes

Total Time: **30** Minutes

INGREDIENTS

- Thyme
- 100 ml beer
- 2 tbs onion powder
- 3 tsp smoked paprika
- 2 limes
- 2 red snappers

DIRECTIONS

1. Mix the seasonings together: thyme, onion powder and paprika
2. Rub the fish with the seasoning and place lime slices inside the snappers
3. Allow to marinate covered for about 1 hour
4. Grill the fish for about 20 minutes on both sides
5. Baste the fish with beer as it cooks

6. Serve drizzled with lime juice

CASHEW CHICKEN

Serves: **6**

Prep Time: **10**   Minutes

Cook Time: **50**   Minutes

Total Time: **60**   Minutes

INGREDIENTS

- 1 lb chicken breasts
- ¼ cup cashews
- 8 oz water chestnuts
- 1 bell pepper
- 1/3 cup orange juice
- 3 tbs soy sauce
- 10 oz mandarin oranges in syrup
- 3 cups brown rice
- ½ cup green onion
- 1 tbs ginger
- 1 cup chicken broth
- 1 ½ tbs cornstarch
- 1 ½ tsp oil

DIRECTIONS

1. Cut the chicken breasts into strips

2. Mix cornstarch and orange juice in a bowl, then add the chicken and cover

3. Allow to marinate for about 1 hour

4. Cook the cashews in hot oil for about 30 seconds

5. Add the chicken mixture to pan and cook until the chicken is a little browned

6. Add the water chestnuts, bell pepper and green onions and cook for 5 more minutes

7. Mix 1 tbs cornstarch, soy sauce, broth and add to chicken mixture

8. Bring to a boil, then reduce the heat and cook until thickened

9. Remove from heat and stir in oranges

10. Serve the rice with chicken over and topped with cashews

CHICKEN PIE

Serves: *8*

Prep Time: *40*   Minutes

Cook Time: *20*   Minutes

Total Time: *60*   Minutes

INGREDIENTS

- 1 onion
- 3 carrots
- 1 parsnip
- 3 cup chicken broth
- 1 cup flour
- 1 cup milk
- ½ cup parsley
- 1 cup green peas
- 1 lb chicken breast
- 2 celery stalks
- 2 red potatoes
- 3 tbs thyme
- 2 sheets dough
- Salt
- Pepper

DIRECTIONS

1. Dice the onion, carrot, parsnip, potatoes and celery
2. Cut the chicken into cubes
3. Cook the onions for about 3 minutes, then add the chicken and cook for another 5 minutes
4. Add the parsnip, potatoes, celery, carrots, peas, and chicken stock to a pot and bring to a boil
5. Reduce the heat and cook covered for 5 minutes
6. Add the flour in a bowl and slowly stir in the milk
7. Pour the flour mixture over the broth and cook for 5 minutes
8. Remove from heat and add thyme, parsley, salt and pepper
9. Place the chicken and vegetables in a baking dish, then pour the broth mixture over
10. Cover with the dough
11. Bake in the preheated oven for 20 minutes at 375F
12. Serve immediately

HONEY SHRIMP

Serves: *4*

Prep Time: *5*   Minutes

Cook Time: *10*   Minutes

Total Time: *15*   Minutes

INGREDIENTS

- 1/3 cup soy sauce
- 3 cloves garlic
- 1/3 cup honey
- 2 tbs ginger
- 1 lb shrimp
- 3 tsp olive oil

DIRECTIONS

1. Mix honey, garlic, soy sauce and ginger together
2. Add the shrimp in and allow to marinate covered for at least 10 minutes in the refrigerator
3. Cook the shrimp in hot oil until done, then remove from skillet
4. Pour the marinade into the skillet and bring to a boil, cooking for 3 minutes

5. Return the shrimp to the skillet and cook 1 more minute

6. Serve immediately

SPAGHETTI PIE

Serves: **16**

Prep Time: **15** Minutes

Cook Time: **35** Minutes

Total Time: **50** Minutes

INGREDIENTS

- ½ cup ricotta
- 1 lb ground beef
- 1/3 cup Parmesan
- 8 oz spaghetti
- 2 eggs

Vegetables:

- 1 onion
- 2 cups broccoli
- 3 garlic cloves
- 2 handfuls spinach
- 6 oz mushrooms
- 2 tbs oregano
- mozzarella
- 2 cups tomato sauce

DIRECTIONS

1. Cook the pasta, then drain
2. Mix eggs, Parmesan and ricotta together
3. Add spaghetti and toss to coat
4. Transfer to a baking pan and press it down
5. Cook the meat until brown, then cook the vegetables until soft
6. Add the beef over the vegetables along with the tomato sauce
7. Spoon the beef mixture over the pasta and sprinkle with mozzarella
8. Bake for about 35 minutes
9. Allow to cool, then cut and serve

TURKEY & BROCCOLI PASTA

Serves: **6**

Prep Time: **10** Minutes

Cook Time: **20** Minutes

Total Time: **30** Minutes

INGREDIENTS

- 12 oz pasta
- 8 oz broccoli
- 3 tbs olive oil
- 15 oz ground turkey
- 2 tsp paprika
- 1 tsp red pepper flakes
- 1 tsp salt
- ½ cup basil
- 1/3 cup Parmesan cheese
- 3 tsp garlic

DIRECTIONS

1. Cook the pasta and add the broccoli in the last 3 minutes of cooking
2. Drain and cover

3. Cook the turkey, garlic, paprika, salt and red pepper flakes in hot oil until browned

4. Add the turkey and basil to the pasta

5. Mix until combined

6. Serve sprinkled with Parmesan cheese

DESSERTS

PEANUT BUTTER COOKIES

Serves: **8**
Prep Time: **5**   Minutes

Cook Time: **10**   Minutes

Total Time: **15**   Minutes

INGREDIENTS

- 1 cup peanut butter
- 1 tsp vanilla
- 1 egg
- 1 cup sugar

DIRECTIONS

1. Mix the ingredients together
2. Form balls from the dough and press them down on a cookie sheet
3. Bake for 10 minutes at 350F
4. Allow to cool, then serve

Serves: *8*

Prep Time: *10*   Minutes

Cook Time: *30*   Minutes

Total Time: *40*   Minutes

INGREDIENTS

Filling:

- 5 cups apples

- 1 ½ tsp lemon juice

- 1 tsp apple pie spice

- 3 tbs sugar

Topping:

- 4 tbs butter

- 1/3 cup sugar

- 3 tbs flour

- ½ cup rolled oats

- 1/3 tsp apple pie spice

- 2 tbs honey

DIRECTIONS

1. Mix the filling ingredients together in a bowl
2. Mix the topping ingredients separately
3. Sprinkle the filling with the topping crumbles
4. Bake for about 30 minutes until golden brown
5. Allow to cool, then serve

CHOCOLATE MOUSSE

Serves: **4**

Prep Time: **10**   Minutes

Cook Time: **30**   Minutes

Total Time: **40**   Minutes

INGREDIENTS

- 1 avocado
- 2 tsp vanilla
- 1/3 cup yogurt
- Sweetener
- 4 tbs coconut milk
- 2 oz chocolate
- 3 tbs cocoa powder

DIRECTIONS

1. Place the ingredients in a blender except for the sweetener
2. Pulse until smooth, then add the sweetener
3. Allow to chill, then serve

LEMON CAKE

Serves: **5**

Prep Time: **10**   Minutes

Cook Time: **90**   Minutes

Total Time: **100**   Minutes

INGREDIENTS

- 9 eggs
- 1 lemon
- 1 ½ cups vegetable shortening
- 2 tsp vanilla
- 2 cups flour
- 3 cups sugar

DIRECTIONS

1. Cream the shortening until smooth
2. Slowly add the sugar in and continue mixing
3. Add one egg at a time mixing after each one, then stir in vanilla and lemon juice
4. Sift the flour and add it to the mixture
5. Pour the batter into a greased tube pan
6. Bake in the preheated oven for 90 minutes at 300F

7. Allow to cool completely and serve

CHEESECAKE BROWNIES

Serves: **10**

Prep Time: **10** Minutes

Cook Time: **20** Minutes

Total Time: **30** Minutes

INGREDIENTS

Brownie:
- 1/3 tsp salt
- ½ cup cocoa powder
- 1 egg
- 1/3 cup milk
- 1 cup Greek yogurt
- ½ cup rolled oats
- ½ cup stevia
- 2 tsp baking powder

Cheesecake:
- 1 egg
- 1/3 cup stevia
- 6 oz cream cheese

Topping:
- 2 tbs chocolate chips

DIRECTIONS

1. Mix Greek yogurt, oats, 1 egg, tagatose, baking powder, milk, cocoa powder and salt together in a bowl

2. Pour the batter into a pan

3. In another bowl, mix 1 egg, cream cheese and 1/3 cup tagatose

4. Pour the cheesecake layer over the brownie mixture

5. Sprinkle chocolate chips over

6. Bake in the preheated oven for 20 minutes at 400F

7. Allow to cool, then serve

PUMPKIN SQUARES

Serves: **24**

Prep Time: **20** Minutes

Cook Time: **40** Minutes

Total Time: **60** Minutes

INGREDIENTS

- 2 cups flour
- 1/3 tsp allspice
- 1 ½ cup walnuts
- 1/3 cup flour
- 2 eggs
- 12 oz pumpkin
- 15 oz condensed milk
- 1/3 cup brown sugar
- 1 cup butter
- 2 tsp cinnamon
- 1/3 tsp salt

DIRECTIONS

1. Mix brown sugar, flour, sugar and butter until crumbly

2. Stir in the walnuts

3. Press the mixture, except for 1 cup, onto the bottom of a baking dish

4. Mix the remaining ingredients together, then pour over the crust and sprinkle with the reserved mixture

5. Bake for at least 40 minutes, until golden brown in the preheated oven at 350F

MINI CHEESECAKES

Serves: **12**

Prep Time: **10**   Minutes

Cook Time: **60**   Minutes

Total Time: **40**   Minutes

INGREDIENTS
Crust:
- 8 graham crackers
- 5 tbs butter
- 3 tbs xylitol

Filling:
- 15 oz cream cheese
- ½ cup xylitol
- 2 tsp vanilla
- ½ cup heavy cream

DIRECTIONS

1. Place the crust ingredients together in a food processor and process until crumbly
2. Divide the mixture into a muffin tray
3. Mix the heavy cream using an electric mixer until firm
4. Separately mix the xylitol, cream cheese and vanilla

5. Add the heavy cream and blend it on low to combine
6. Divide the mixture over the crust in the muffin tray
7. Allow to set in the refrigerator for at least 1 hour
8. Serve topped with berries

PEANUT BUTTER DESSERT

Serves: *16*
Prep Time: *10* Minutes

Cook Time: *5*   Minutes

Total Time: *15* Minutes

INGREDIENTS

- 15 oz chickpeas
- 2 tbs honey
- 3 tbs milk
- 1/3 cup peanut butter

DIRECTIONS

1. Place the ingredients except for the milk in a blender
2. Pulse until smooth
3. Gradually add the milk and continue to pulse until smooth
4. Serve with fruits or cookies

STRAWBERRY CHEESECAKE

Serves: *8*

Prep Time: *5*   Minutes

Cook Time: *10*   Minutes

Total Time: *15*   Minutes

INGREDIENTS

- ½ cup cream cheese
- 3 tsp lemon juice
- 1/3 cup strawberry preserves
- 4 dates
- 1/3 cup Greek yogurt
- 3 tbs sugar
- 1 cup strawberries
- ¼ cum almonds

DIRECTIONS

1. Using an electric mixer, mix together yogurt, sugar, cream cheese and lemon juice
2. Separately combine the strawberries and preserves
3. Pulse the almonds until crumb consistency, then add dates and pulse until combined

4. Divide the almond mixture among 8 dessert dishes, then top with yogurt mixture, strawberries and then repeat

5. Serve cold

FAST FRUIT SALAD

Serves: **2**

Prep Time: **5**   Minutes

Cook Time: **5**   Minutes

Total Time: **10**   Minutes

INGREDIENTS

- ½ tsp cinnamon
- 3 tbs roasted almonds
- 1 cup mango
- 1/3 cup yogurt
- 1 ½ cup strawberries

DIRECTIONS

1. Mix everything together in a bowl to coat the fruits in yogurt
2. Add cinnamon
3. Serve topped with sliced almonds

SMOOTHIES

PEANUT BUTTER SMOOTHIE

Serves: *1*
Prep Time: 5   Minutes
Cook Time: 5   Minutes
Total Time: *10*   Minutes

INGREDIENTS

- 1 tsp vanilla
- 1/3 cup milk
- 1/3 cup Greek yogurt
- 1 cup ice
- 2 tbs peanut butter
- 1 banana

DIRECTIONS

1. In a blender place all ingredients and blend until smooth
2. Pour smoothie in a glass and serve

PINEAPPLE SMOOTHIE

Serves: **1**
Prep Time: **5**   Minutes

Cook Time: **5**   Minutes

Total Time: **10**   Minutes

INGREDIENTS

- 1/3 cup almond milk
- ½ cup carrots
- 2 tbs oats
- 1/3 cup yogurt
- ½ cup pineapple juice
- 1 banana
- 1 cup berries
- 1 ½ cup spinach leaves
- 1 cup strawberries
- 3 tbs flax seed
- 2 tbs chia seeds
- 1 cup ice

DIRECTIONS

1. In a blender place all ingredients and blend until smooth
2. Pour smoothie in a glass and serve

5 INGREDIENTS SMOOTHIE

Serves: *1*
Prep Time: *5*   Minutes

Cook Time: *5*   Minutes

Total Time: *10*   Minutes

INGREDIENTS

- 1 ½ cups orange juice
- ½ cup yogurt
- 1 tbs sugar
- 1 banana
- 1 ½ cups berries

DIRECTIONS

1. In a blender place all ingredients and blend until smooth
2. Pour smoothie in a glass and serve

STRAWBERRY SMOOTHIE

Serves: *1*

Prep Time: *5*   Minutes

Cook Time: *5*   Minutes

Total Time: *10*   Minutes

INGREDIENTS

- 1 cup yogurt
- 1/3 cup skim milk
- 1 banana
- ½ cup strawberries

DIRECTIONS

1. In a blender place all ingredients and blend until smooth
2. Pour smoothie in a glass and serve

MANGO SMOOTHIE

Serves: *1*

Prep Time: *5*   Minutes

Cook Time: *5*   Minutes

Total Time: *10* Minutes

INGREDIENTS

- 1 cup coconut water
- 5 tbs orange juice
- 1 cup ice
- 1 cup Greek yogurt
- 1 cup mango

DIRECTIONS

1. In a blender place all ingredients and blend until smooth
2. Pour smoothie in a glass and serve

SPINACH SMOOTHIE

Serves: **1**

Prep Time: **5**   Minutes

Cook Time: **5**   Minutes

Total Time: **10**   Minutes

INGREDIENTS

- 1/3 cup milk
- 1/3 cup Greek yogurt
- 2 tbs butter
- 1 banana
- 1/3 cup strawberries
- 1/3 cup spinach

DIRECTIONS

1. In a blender place all ingredients and blend until smooth
2. Pour smoothie in a glass and serve

OATS SMOOTHIE

Serves: *1*

Prep Time: *5*   Minutes

Cook Time: *5*   Minutes

Total Time: *10*   Minutes

INGREDIENTS

- 1 banana
- 10 strawberries
- ½ cup oats
- 1 ½ tbs flaxseed
- 1 cup skim milk
- 1 tsp vanilla
- 2 tsp honey

DIRECTIONS

1. In a blender place all ingredients and blend until smooth
2. Pour smoothie in a glass and serve

BERRY BEAN SMOOTHIE

Serves: *1*
Prep Time: *5*   Minutes

Cook Time: *5*   Minutes

Total Time: *10*   Minutes

INGREDIENTS

- 2 cup orange juice
- 2 tsp cinnamon
- 2 cups strawberries
- 4 tbs honey
- ¼ tsp nutmeg
- 1 cup ice
- 15 oz beans

DIRECTIONS

1. In a blender place all ingredients and blend until smooth
2. Pour smoothie in a glass and serve

ORANGE SMOOTHIE

Serves: *1*

Prep Time: *5*   Minutes

Cook Time: *5*   Minutes

Total Time: *10* Minutes

INGREDIENTS

- 2 oranges
- 1 cup ice
- 3 tsp vanilla
- 1 banana
- ½ cup milk

DIRECTIONS

1. In a blender place all ingredients and blend until smooth
2. Pour smoothie in a glass and serve

BLUEBERRIES SMOOTHIE

Serves: *1*

Prep Time: *5*   Minutes

Cook Time: *5*   Minutes

Total Time: *10*   Minutes

INGREDIENTS

- 1 cup ice
- 3 tbs avocado
- 2 tbs chia seeds
- 1/3 cup milk
- ½ cup cauliflower
- 1 cup blueberries

DIRECTIONS

1. In a blender place all ingredients and blend until smooth
2. Pour smoothie in a glass and serve

THANK YOU FOR READING THIS BOOK!

Printed in Great Britain
by Amazon